28 SECRETS to GLOW UP

Tips for Health, Energy and Radiance

By Marianne Talkovski, L.Ac, LE

Copyright © 2020 by Marianne Talkovski

All rights reserved. No part of this publication may be reproduced, distributed or transmitted in any form or by any means, including photocopying, recording, or other electronic or mechanical methods, without the prior written permission of the author, except in the case of brief quotations embodied in critical reviews and certain other noncommercial uses permitted by copyright law. For permission requests, contact the author at: www.mariannetalkovski.com

28 Secrets to Glow Up/Marianne Talkovski

ISBN 978-0-578-79906-3

For Jasmine, King of the Flowers.

*Always remember to love
who you see in the mirror.*

Contents

FOREWORD BY SUSAN HYATT............................... 9

INTRODUCTION.. 11

SECRET #1 FROM RAISINS TO GRAPES...................... 15

SECRET #2 TAKE OUT THE TRASH 18

SECRET #3 THE MORE FLOW, THE MORE GLOW 20

SECRET #4 THE ULTIMATE QI BOOST...................... 25

SECRET #5 BEAUTY SLEEP 28

SECRET #6 ENERGY ELIXIR............................... 32

SECRET #7 DRINK YOUR SOLIDS, CHEW YOUR LIQUIDS 34

SECRET #8 CHOOSE YOUR FUEL........................... 38

SECRET #9 ALKALINITY: THE SOLUTION TO THE ROOT OF ALL EVIL ... 42

SECRET #10 DIGESTIVE FIRE 46

SECRET #11 ALL ROADS LEAD TO THE FACE 50

SECRET #12 MAGIC BUTTONS 53

SECRET #13 TWERK IT 58

SECRET #14 PARK IT.................................... 60

SECRET #15 PRESENCE 64

SECRET #16 CHILL PILL 69

SECRET #17 BEING 74

SECRET #18 THE BOUNCER 77

SECRET #19	2 WAY STREET 82
SECRET #20	LET GO, LET FLOW 89
SECRET #21	THE GOLDEN NUGGET 94
SECRET #22	THE BAMBOO TREE 100
SECRET #23	THE DIVINE DOWNLOAD 105
SECRET #24	THE GARDEN 111
SECRET #25	DIAMOND GLOW 117
SECRET #26	AN ATTITUDE OF GRATITUDE 121
SECRET #27	SILENCE IS GOLDEN 125
SECRET #28	KISS YOURSELF 129

A SELF-CARE MANIFESTO 133

RESOURCES. 134

ACKNOWLEDGEMENTS 135

NEXT STEPS. 137

ABOUT MARIANNE 139

THANK YOU! 141

Foreword by Susan Hyatt
Master certified life coach | shyatt.com
Founder of Bare for women and Bold for girls

Are you tired? Most women that I know are completely exhausted. Physically tired. Mentally depleted. Living with a weariness that no amount of espresso can cure.

As women, as a collective, why are we so tired? Why don't we feel good? Well, you don't have to be a rocket scientist to figure out why.

If you spend your days:

- Dieting and obsessively tracking what you eat.
- Worrying that your body isn't thin, tight, or smooth enough.
- Consuming media that makes you feel worse about yourself.
- Bullying yourself with negative thoughts about your appearance and your life.
- Over-working, over-scheduling, and creating a never-ending cycle of busyness.
- Behaving like your family's personal maid, chef, chauffeur, tutor, and therapist.
- Giving excessive amounts of your time, energy, and resources

to others (your boss, clients, kids, spouse) while neglecting your own needs.
- Putting your health on the very bottom of your priority list (if it even makes it onto the list at all...)

Is that what you're doing, most days? Is that what your life looks like? Then you are going to feel exhausted. It's inevitable. Now is the time to break the cycle of tiredness, self-neglect, and poor health. Now is the time to get serious about self-care and decide, "I will be a woman who takes excellent care of herself."

As you make the shift into this new way of being, you will need a loving, compassionate guide—a woman who has "been there" and who "gets it." Marianne is one of the finest guides I could imagine.

Marianne is a passionate entrepreneur. She's a coach certified in working with women and girls on body image and health issues. She's a mother who is determined to be a positive role model for her daughter. She has been on her own health journey, to hell and back, and she brings all of these perspectives to you.

Enjoy this beautiful book. Let it inspire you to Glow Up and start taking better care of yourself every day.

You only get one body. Give it love. Your body is your home for your entire life, and it's the only one you get, so treat it like you would treat anything that is precious to you. That same tenderness and care that you would give to a newborn baby, or anyone else that you love, give it to yourself. This book will show you the way.

- Susan

Introduction

Welcome to 28 Secrets to Glow Up! In this book, you will discover a variety of healthy, easy tips and little doses of luxurious rituals to get glowing skin, radiant energy, a pep in your step and a smile in your heart. It was written as a manual to absorb in bite-size pieces so you can incorporate what resonates with you into your daily habits. There are journal prompts sprinkled throughout the book as well to capture and speak your thoughts into existence. I recommend trying each secret once and notice what makes you feel good. When you feel good, it shows, which is a must to Glow Up.

I want to honor you for prioritizing and investing time and energy into your self-care. Even just picking up this book is an act of self-love.

There are a few core messages embedded into each tip:

- **You can be an advocate for your own health.** No one will know your body better than you do – no doctor, therapist, healer or even lover. Listen to your body. Take care of it. The secrets in this book are a great way to build habits that help you feel good on the inside and outside.

- **You can age with grace and grit.** You are not destined to become insignificant as you get older; in fact, you can become more radiant when your self-care habits become non-negotiable. It is possible to live a long life full of health, energy, love and adventures!

- **When you love yourself when you see yourself, you not only elevate your self-esteem, but you also elevate humanity.** It may sound corny or cliché, but just know that the thoughts you think and the things you say to yourself have a direct impact on your energy and radiance.

- **Self-care is the winning strategy to sustain your energy, and ultimately, to get your glow on.** You may feel that you don't have enough time or money to invest in yourself. If this is something that comes up for you often, I want you to know that it's not that you don't have enough time or money, it's that you don't have enough energy. Energy is a force of power to get things done. If you feel depleted, overwhelmed or exhausted and find yourself running non-stop on empty, it is critical that you focus on:

    Restoring
    Building
    Protecting
    Nourishing and
    Conserving your energy

Your energy is your most important resource. Without further ado, let's get glowing!

My story

I wrote this book for a variety of reasons. First and foremost, I want my daughter to grow up knowing these secrets so she can learn to manage and protect her energy through self-care strategies. It is my intention that she learns to radically love herself at a very young age, so it is ingrained in her that accepting yourself is healthy. I also want my clients to have a manual they can reference based on our work together that contains simple do-able steps with quick wins. Finally, I want my colleagues to have a tool to share with their clients that could support their work as well. It is important to me that as many people as possible have a positive resource on body image, healthy aging, and healthcare.

I grew up as the daughter of a Filipina immigrant and an American sailor. My mother wanted me to be accepted as an American, so unfortunately I did not learn to speak Tagalog. I went to schools with predominantly white kids, so I often felt like I was an outsider with my almond eyes, dark hair, olive skin and curvy build. Growing up, I received messages that I needed to be a size 4 or 6 to fit in or to be considered popular. I was told that if I lost 15 pounds, I would be prettier (diet) and in order to be successful I needed to work really hard (hustle). I constantly thought that I needed to know more before I was enough (hustle) and that I had to look a certain way to be accepted (diet).

This sparked a cascade of events:

- I never had senior class photos taken
- I second-guessed my knowledge, abilities, talents and skills constantly

- I hid from public recognition and passed up many opportunities for growth
- I battled with bulimia between the ages of 14-24
- I worked myself into stage 3 adrenal exhaustion by age 31
- I walked away unscathed (thankfully) from a semi totaling my car while driving 65 mph in a mad dash to over-service clients and seek validation outside of myself
- I struggled with fertility challenges for a year before conceiving my healthy daughter

Despite all of these challenges, I managed to pursue an education in esthetics and Chinese Medicine. I learned ancient secrets for longevity, health and beauty. I also pursued 5 different life and health coaching certifications and training in leadership. In 2018, after getting clear on my purpose and which passion to pursue, I boldly declared in front of my leadership cohort that I wanted to be an example of healthy aging and shift the current paradigm on healthcare, body image, diversity and our pervasive type A work culture. The facilitator of the group was a man in his 60s. He challenged me by saying that he couldn't see people listening to an early 30 something teach about healthy aging, to which I replied, "well that's exactly my point, because tomorrow I turn 40".

And now I want to share my tips, secrets and gems that have helped me radically love and accept my body to age gracefully with radiant energy with you.

Secret #1
From Raisins To Grapes

"If there is magic on this planet, it is contained in water."

LOREN EISELEY

My husband refers to raisins as "shrunk grapes". It's funny that he calls them that because obviously that is exactly what they are and that is what I often tell my clients to picture when we talk about hydration. Dehydrated skin looks like raisins and does not glow.

Many times, I hear my clients say they feel their skin is extremely dry, even if they drink tons of water. There are a number of reasons why this can happen – change in seasons, exposure to air conditioning or heaters, travel, excessive sweating or even deficiencies in vitamins, minerals and electrolytes. I also explain that just because you drink tons of water doesn't mean the skin will benefit to the degree that other organ systems will benefit. In fact, the skin is the furthest organ from the digestive organs and is affected by changes in our environment constantly; therefore, it is vital that we support our skin with topical hydration.

When people tell me that they don't like wrinkles, I explain to them that if they spread a wrinkle and it disappears, it most likely has not set in the dermal layer which means they are suffering from dehydration. If you add hydration into the skin, it plumps the skin from looking like a raisin to looking like a grape.

I recommend using topical and internal hyaluronic acid (HA) to effectively deliver hydration in the skin. I suggest using HA derived from sources like marine algae or marshmallow root because they are plant-based. Hyaluronic acid holds moisture in our tissues and our joints. It's important to supplement this into our skin because after age 25, we start to produce an enzyme called hyaluronidase that breaks hyaluronic acid down. This creates dehydration not only in our skin, but internally as well.

I start every morning with a cup of hot water and squeeze ½ a lemon into it. I also add a scoop of tasteless, odorless Whole Body Collagen Powder (currently I love the version from Designs For Health). Lemons are acidic outside of the body, but when ingested, they become alkaline and flush the liver and kidneys (stay tuned for more on alkalinity in a future secret). I find when I start my mornings this way, I feel hydrated, clean and energetic.

Action Step #1 *start your day off with a cup of lemon water. Optional: add collagen and/or hyaluronic acid powder. Drink this every day for the next 30 days and revel in the results.*

Action Step #2 *consult with your esthetician on a topical hyaluronic acid that will plump your skin. See the resources section for my favorite skincare line recommendation.*

Secret #2
Take Out The Trash

"If you have no time for health, health has no time for you."

JUSTIN ZHENG JIXIN

Did you know that your body has a system that acts as a natural garbage disposal? Yes, we naturally detox through our breath, urine, bowels, and sweat, but we also detox through our lymphatic system. Detoxing is important to clean out our bodies by removing toxins, cellular waste, environmental toxins and pathogens that can create imbalances with our hormones.

The lymphatic system is a network of vessels and other tissues that maintains fluid balance and fights infection through detoxification. The lymphatic system transports lymph, a fluid containing infection-fighting white blood cells, throughout the body. Lymph only moves in one direction, toward the heart. Your lymphatic system doesn't have a pump and relies on muscle motion to improve circulation. If you don't exercise regularly, your lymph can stagnate, leading to frequent colds, fatigue, brain fog, inflammation, skin breakouts, or even mood swings.

That's why I recommend dry brushing. When you dry brush, your lymph fluid carries waste products and destroyed bacteria back into the bloodstream. The liver or kidneys then remove these from the blood. The body passes them out with other body waste, through bowel movements or urine. Dry-brushing is a simple, affordable ancient practice to boost your lymph system and exfoliate your skin. It helps eliminate toxic build up on the surface of the skin and increases lymphatic drainage. Other benefits of dry brushing may include smooth clear skin, the reduced appearance of cellulite, and a short-term energy boost.

Try it before your shower so you can rinse off any dead cells afterwards.

To dry brush your skin, grab a natural-bristle brush with a long handle so you can reach your back. Start from your feet and brush upward toward your heart in long strokes. It can be sensitive on the abdomen, breasts and neck, so lighten up pressure as needed.

Action Step: *Get a natural-bristle brush and start each morning with a dry brush routine for the next 30 days.*

Secret #3
The More Flow, The More Glow

"I regret taking such good care of my skin."

SAID NO ONE EVER

One of the things that I like to share with my clients is that radiance comes from healthy blood flow. It's important to cultivate healthy circulation because blood carries oxygen and vital nutrients that are broken down from our food to our tissues. Exercise is one way to boost our circulation, and there are other ways too!

Cooking with spices like ginger, paprika, cinnamon, and turmeric is a great way to increase metabolism. These spices can even be found in some innovative skincare products* (see **A word about skincare products** below) to help boost circulation, offering oxygenation, detoxification and better absorption of products to the face.

Another great way to boost blood flow is massage. Now I know that massaging yourself is not the same as getting a massage; however, gua sha, facial rolling and cupping are fantastic ways to massage your face and neck, among many other benefits. Also, approximately 30% of our lymph nodes are located in our face and neck. Note: if you identify as male and are reading this, I encourage and invite you to take care of your skin too! I know the media targets women primarily in the beauty industry, which is odd to me considering men have skin too.

There are a few tools made from gemstones with varying metaphysical properties, so I recommend choosing what speaks most to you. Jade is often used for cooling the skin and is known as the stone of eternal youth, Rose Quartz is used for soothing the skin and is known as the stone of self-love and Amethyst is used for calming the skin and is known as the stone of peace. I recommend the following:

- Facial rolling for reducing puffiness, increasing product penetration and soothing the skin

- Gua Sha for relieving facial and jaw tension, lifting and contouring the skin and manual lymphatic drainage

- Cupping for increased circulation, relieving muscle tension and stimulating cellular repair

I love my tools from Mount Lai and Wildling (see the resource page for discounts). Here is a diagram to help learn how to use your tools. I recommend using these daily for optimal results.

Action Step: *Invest in a gua sha or facial rolling tool and add this to your skincare routine once a day.*

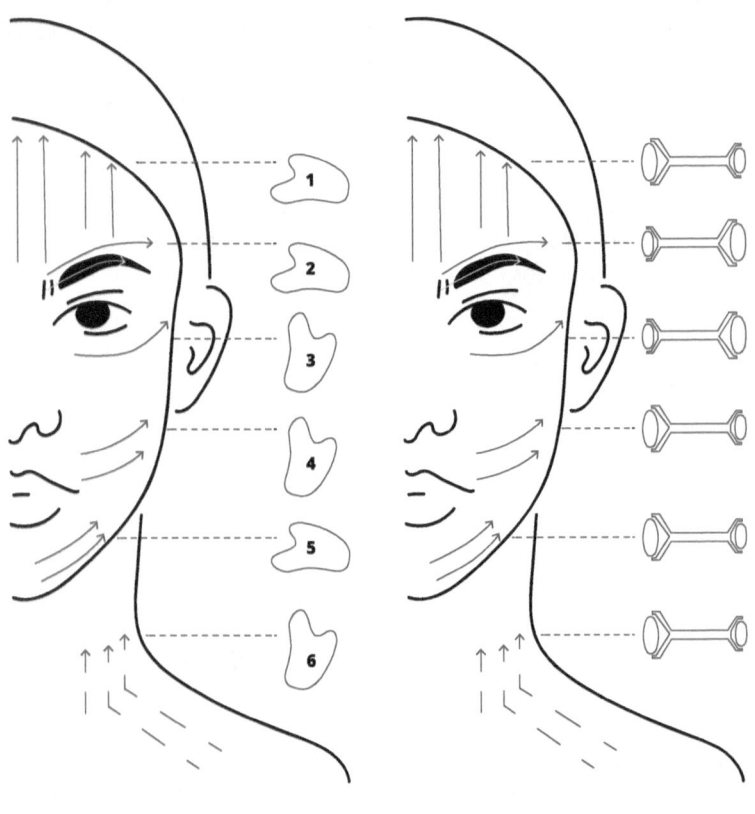

Follow the arrows a minimum of 3-4 passes with your tool to guide lymph, lift and sculpt tissue and get that glow!

A word about skincare products

I work with a range of clientele – from women who love all sorts of products, women who feel guilty about purchasing anything for themselves, men who secretly take care of their skin, to men who completely avoid any kind of skincare altogether. In my lifestyle, skincare is non-negotiable – it makes my skin feel good, look good and it also reminds me to take exquisite care of myself. There's something so nourishing about investing in a special product to support you aesthetically. To me, it says, I am proud of my skin and want to take care if it.

There are so many products on the market and in a $532 billion dollar industry (as of 2019), it can be overwhelming what to choose and where to start. Here are a few recommendations to get that glow:

- Choose clean natural and organic products void of parabens, sulfates, chemicals, mineral oil, artificial coloring and synthetic dyes or fragrances, petroleum jelly or any other multi-syllabic words that you can't pronounce that aren't from a natural source.

- Invest in exfoliants, masks and serums. These are the game-changers of a skincare line. People will typically purchase cleansers and moisturizers, and these product categories will maintain their skin, but they will not change the skin. You need the medicine – the serums —for ultimate lasting effects. Serums are formulated with a tiny molecular structure to provide deeper penetration to the living layers of the skin, where change can take place. Exfoliants are important because they help absorption of all following products and they smooth texture and encourage cellular turnover by sloughing off dead skin cells and dirt on the surface of the skin. I always tell my clients "if you want to fertilize your lawn, you have to rake the leaves." Serums are your fertilizer, exfoliants are the rake.

- There are other steps to a routine. Having a routine creates compounding results over time. I recommend consulting with a professional to consider your skin type, concerns and your preferences. Prevention and maintenance are easier than correction, so the sooner you start caring for your skin, the better. Due to the nature of this book, these are tiny do-able suggestions, and there is so much more that can be said. Schedule a facial with a trusted professional for customized recommendations.

Secret #4
The Ultimate Qi Boost

"Breathing is the first act of life, and the last."

JOSEPH H. PILATES

According to Chinese Medicine, Qi (pronounced chee or chi) is the source of our energy. Qi is cultivated through our breath and food. While eating is a voluntary exercise, breathing is not. Fortunately, our bodies are designed to breathe on their own, without us needing to remember to do so.

Here's something that we don't consider: the quality of Qi does not simply depend on what we breathe in or what we eat. The quality of Qi also depends on how we breathe and how we eat. Which means that when we are conscious of taking in full, deep inhales and releasing full, lengthy exhales, the quality of our Qi improves. Our energy improves.

There are a variety of breath work practices that I walk my clients through when they come in for acupuncture. I recommend you try each one for a day to see what your body, mind and spirit respond well too:

THE 4-7-8 BREATH

I love this practice because it's a great way to calm the nervous system down, it can be practiced anywhere and it's free!

Take an inhale for a 4 count, hold for a 7 count and release for an 8 count. Practice this breath 3 times and invite your mind to connect to your body by slowing down.

THE 4-4-6-4 BREATH

I love this practice for reducing mental chatter because it really allows you to notice the time between breaths, when inhales become exhales and exhales become inhales. Take an inhale for a 4 count, hold that inhale for 4 counts, release your exhale for 6 counts and then hold the bottom of that exhale for 4 counts. I remind my clients that breathing is a cycle that is a microcosm of other cycles – the inhale comes in and flows out just like digestion flows in and elimination flows out or ocean waves flow in and out. Notice the pause between the transitions, no matter how subtle that may be. When we notice the transition or the time between breaths, we begin to appreciate what is to come versus moving on to the next thing without awareness. Practice this four times to increase mindfulness and presence.

THREE-PART BREATH

I love this practice for activating energy in our core. Imagine your belly is a balloon. Inhale and fill the balloon in your low belly. As you exhale pull up your 'bathroom muscles' and lift the balloon up and behind your belly button. Practice this twice more. Then, with your next inhale, imagine the balloon is expanding from the low belly, out through the sides of your rib cage. Again, with your exhale, pull up your bathroom muscles up and behind your belly button. Practice this twice more. Finally, with your next inhale, imagine the balloon is expanding from the low belly, out through the sides of your rib cage and up to your collar bones. With your exhale, lift your bathroom muscles up and behind your belly button. Practice this twice more. Return to normal breathing.

ALTERNATE NOSTRIL BREATHING

This is such a great practice for creating balance in your brain. If you are feeling too logical and needing a creative boost or if you are doing a lot of dreaming and not doing, this breath practice helps to unite the left and right hemispheres of your brain. Close the right nostril with your right thumb. Exhale through your left nostril. Inhale through your left nostril. Close your left nostril with your right ring finger. Open your right nostril and exhale. Inhale through your right nostril and close. Open your left nostril and exhale. Repeat this cycle for 10 breaths. Release your hand in your lap.

Action Step: *practice each breath for 7 days straight first thing in the morning before getting out of bed. Notice how you feel after each breath practice.*

Secret #5
Beauty Sleep

"Sleep is the best meditation."

DALAI LAMA

Did you know that when you sleep, you heal? Sleep is the time for our bodies to restore, our minds to rest and our hearts to be at peace. It has been medicine for me after intense physical exertion, excessive studying and tragic breakups. When I'm feeling troubled about something, I rely on sleep for my body to heal and for my mind to gain clarity. When my daughter was born, my husband and I purchased a special bassinet that would rock her to sleep because I refused to be a mom who was sleep-deprived and struggling throughout the day. There was a considerable investment up front of $870, but she slept soundly for 10 months, which averaged approximately $3 per day. That $3 dollars a day was well worth it for my sanity!

In Chinese Medicine, the Heart is the organ that governs sleep. The spirit resides in the Heart. When our sleep is disturbed, our spirit is disturbed. In turn, when our spirit is disturbed, our sleep is often disturbed as well. This is why it is so important to cultivate sleep hygiene. These days, many clients share with me they use their smartphones as alarm clocks. Which means they have a small computer buzzing with radiation and electricity right next to their beds and heads. I used to do this as well, until I was given the recommendation by writer Alexandra Franzen to create a charging station for all of my electronics in a separate room. This has revolutionized my sleep. I am not tempted to peek at my phone if I wake up in the middle of the night to use the restroom. I sleep through the night more soundly. And I'm not worried about my brain not fully turning off.

There are other things you can do to safeguard your sleep. Purchase black out curtains. Remove all sources of light that can't be turned off. Take any plants out of your bedroom (growth is the energy of plants, which can be too stimulating for your rest). Watch tv in your living room and reserve your bedroom for sleep and sex. Clean off your nightstand. Adopt a nighttime ritual of drinking a calming tea to help you to settle in for the night that will ultimately set you up for success the next day.

If you remember your dreams, keep a journal on your nightstand to write them down. Your dreams carry messages about you and your life. If you are troubled about something, ask yourself a question before laying down to rest, and invite your dreams to provide solutions. When you wake up fully rested, it shows in your spirit.

Action Step: *Create a charging station with all electronics outside of your bedroom. Two hours before you go to sleep, sip on a calming tea. Reflect on your day before sleeping by asking the following questions:*

What did I learn today?

What was delightful for me?

Before you fall asleep and possibly dream, ask yourself "what does spirit want me to know?"

Secret #6 – Energy Elixir

"You can't enjoy life if you're not nourishing your body."

TRACEY GOLD

One of the things that I learned during my Chinese Medical training is that bone broth is incredibly nourishing and healing for digestion and immunity. The Chinese believe that our energy and immunity are housed in our gut. Whenever one of my clients feels under the weather or a cold coming on, I recommend they cook a batch of the following and sip on it all day long:

- Juice from 1 lemon
- 1 clove of minced garlic
- 1 tsp minced ginger
- 1-2 sprigs of thyme
- ½ tsp of Dulse or Kelp seaweed or sprig of Kombu
- 1 chopped stalk of scallion
- Bone broth from bison / turkey / beef or chicken (I like The

Flavorful Chef brand but you can also make your own broth with high-quality bones and 2 tbsp apple cider vinegar to help leach the minerals out of the bones)
- ¼ tsp of miso – optional* *(add after removing liquid from heat)*
- 1 tsp of honey *(add after removing liquid from heat)*

You can get creative and add additional ingredients like a whipped egg, shiitake mushrooms, goji berries, astragalus or red dates. You can freeze the broth and use it as a base for other broths, to cook with your grains or to sip as a tea.

All of these ingredients are antibacterial and immune boosting. I started sipping on this daily and having something warm in my belly to start my mornings has given me an incredible boost in my energy. Consistency is key!

Action step: *Drink this broth daily for 30 days to proactively boost your immunity and observe how your energy levels shift.*

*omit if sensitive to soy

Secret #7
Drink Your Solids, Chew Your Liquids

"You are what you eat, so don't be fast, cheap, easy or fake."

UNKNOWN

In the previous secret, we talked about how our Qi, or life energy, is cultivated through our breath and nutrition. Digestion is one of the hardest processes our bodies go through, and yet, in order for our bodies to function healthfully, we need a variety of nutrients, vitamins and minerals. Like the breath, it is important that we are mindful not only of what we take in as information (oxygen or food), but also how we take it in. So often I hear my patients share they skip meals, eat on the go, eat while standing, or shovel their food down without chewing properly.

Did you know that we produce an enzyme in our saliva when we chew? Amylase is the enzyme that breaks down carbohydrates. When we chew thoroughly, we optimize the process of digestion. We make it easier for our bodies to process and eliminate. Remember, our stomachs do not have teeth.

With your next meal, I invite you to sit down. Set your table with flowers, candles or anything else that would allow you to fully enjoy your experience. Take out your nice dishes and cutlery. Pull out your cloth napkins. Plate your food artfully on your dish and let your eyes feast on the beauty before you. Smell your food. Take in all of the aromas. Notice the temperature. Listen to your fork or spoon clink against your plate or bowl. Take a small bite. Put your fork or spoon down. Close your eyes. Chew each morsel thoroughly. Practice this for the first three bites to truly savor the flavor of your meal.

It is not advised to drink liquids during meals because it can hinder optimal digestion by flushing away enzymes, the catalysts that break food down. When you do drink, hydrate an hour before and after meals, and drink slowly. Imagine if you are drinking a smoothie that you still need to break down the nutrients, so rather than gulp your liquids down, take your time with digesting them as well. Chewing is not only essential to digestion, it is a game changer when it comes to improving it.

Finally, notice what you are taking in when eating. I remember hearing a story about a Chinese businessman who would schedule his important meetings at lunch. After the meal, he would monitor his digestion. If he felt good, he knew it was a good deal. If his digestion was off, he knew it was a bad one. This is a great story to exemplify that we absorb thoughts just like we absorb our food. If you are watching the news while eating, scrolling on your phone, engaging in an upsetting conversation or even reading, it can have an impact on our digestion. Treat your mealtime as sacred and be conscious of what your senses are taking in that could help or hinder your energy.

Action Step: *Set your table as if you are going on a date, with yourself. Choose your favorite place setting, cutlery, dinnerware and set the scene with flowers, candles and music. Invite all of your senses in. Practice the Mindful Eating meditation at www.mariannetalkovski.com/glowup. Close your eyes and chew thoroughly for your first 5 bites. After each bite, set your utensil down and fully savor the flavors of your meal. Continue chewing thoroughly for the remainder of your meal.*

What did you notice about your food?

How did your body feel before, during and after the meal?

_____

_____

_____

_____

_____

_____

_____

_____

Secret #8 – Choose Your Fuel

"To nourish is to flourish."

UNKNOWN

So far we've covered many tips to increase your radiant energy, health and beauty. One of the building blocks to boosting Qi is getting healthy nourishment through food. There is a ton of information circulating on diets and I have tried many of them. I've tried Weight Watchers, South Beach, Keto, Paleo, low calorie, meal replacements, plant-based and many more. What I've discovered is that in order to see consistent results, one must adopt an eating plan that is sustainable.

For me, I need simplicity, ease, strength and pleasure with my eating plan. Since becoming a BARE certified coach*, one of the guidelines I've taken for nourishment is to ask my body "what feels like love?" and in that exploration I check in with myself on if I need food to give me strength and energy (power) or food to give me delight (pleasure). Since looking at food as **information** that gives me energy and can either provide power or pleasure, it has helped me eat what I want, when I want, with attentiveness versus guilt and restriction. It has also freed up so much space mentally for me to focus on making power moves in my life rather than obsessing about calories and pounds.

Whether you have been influenced by diet culture or not, take some time to check in with yourself about what your body needs. Do you need power or pleasure? What foods give you power? What foods give you pleasure? For me, I love chocolate, chips and wine for pleasure and eggs, fish, and nuts for power. Some foods can be categorized as both; for example, I love a cup of my husband's turmeric rice for power and pleasure. It can vary at any given moment, which is why checking in before you get voraciously hungry is ideal.

Action Step: *Choose a minimum of 10 power foods and 10 pleasure foods that feel like love to your body and note them on the following page:*

POWER FOODS

PLEASURE FOODS

_____

_____

_____

_____

_____

_____

_____

_____

_____

_____

_____

_____

_____

_____

*BARE is not a weight-loss plan. It's a 7 Step Program to Transform Your Body, Get More Energy, Feel Amazing, and Become the Bravest, Most Unstoppable Version of You developed by my coach and mentor Susan Hyatt. This tip is a snippet of the BARE process. To inquire more, check out my program New You By Design at www.mariannetalkovski.com/coaching

Secret #9
Alkalinity: The Solution To The Root Of All Evil

"A healthy outside starts from the inside."

ROBERT URICH

In my studies, especially regarding nutrition and skincare, I came to learn what the root of all imbalances, sickness and evil is. It causes issues in our tissues. It expresses itself differently in all of us – whether it's irritation (felt or not felt), pain or discomfort (tiny or colossal), swelling (seen or unseen) or degradation (health or beauty in the mind, body, or spirit) – it lurks and spreads at a cellular level, increasing over time. This evil that exists is known as inflammation.

In medical terms, inflammation presents as heat, swelling, pain or redness.

In Chinese Medicine, it is believed that inflammation or dis-ease can be prompted either through external or internal evils. External evils are physical traumas, injuries or accidents. They can also be climate specific. There are six external evils that pertain to climate: cold, dryness, dampness or humidity, wind, heat and summer-heat. For example, if you move to the desert, and you only experience heat or dryness for the majority of the year, it may create imbalances depending on your constitution and patterns. A Chinese Medical practitioner can help assess this for you during a visit.

Internal evils are prompted through nutrition and our emotions. Inflammation is linked to having an excess level of acidity in our bodies. Every food has a pH level and falls on a spectrum of acidity-alkalinity. When we eat foods that are excessively acidic, it starts to affect the pH levels of our blood because the acidity in our cells has increased. In the skincare world, a new word is trending called "inflamma-ging". This play on words helps to understand that when our bodies are acidic, we tend to age more rapidly.

I had shared this with a client in my early years of practice when I was working in a community style clinic. I remember I had shared with her how she could improve her health by shifting to a more alkaline diet. A month later, she came back to the clinic. When I bent down to read her pulses and chat with her about her focus for that day's treatment, I thought she was a new patient. She asked me "Do you remember me? You told me about the acid-alkaline chart a month ago". She then proceeded to tell me how she made her own flash cards of foods that were alkaline and focused on incorporating those into her diet for the last month. She shared how her energy, mood, digestion and sleep improved. The one thing I noticed that made her unrecognizable was something in her eyes. It was clarity. Her Shen, referred to as spirit in Chinese Medicine, was so clear that it radiated in her face and through her eyes. There was a sense of peace and calm in her presence. She raved about the changes in her energy levels, health, mood and appearance and it was evident in her glowing smile.

Action Step: *Refer to the mini acid-alkaline chart on the following page and make a commitment to eat 80% alkaline / 20% acidic for the next 30 days.*

Note: you can find more extensive charts online if you are looking for a specific food

Add the Alkaline Power Shot to your mornings:

Alkaline Power Shot – for ultimate hormone balancing and alkalizing

- 1 scoop green powder – I love Mighty Maca (see resources)
- ½ a lemon wedge
- 1 shot glass Fire Cider apple cider vinegar or your preferred choice of ACV
- Mix well and drink

ALKALINITY CHEAT SHEET

VEGETABLES

HIGHLY ALKALINE

Low Carb
- Beet Greens
- Cucumber
- Kelp and other sea vegetables
- Maca
- Parsley
- Spinach
- Sprouts, all types
- Alkaline Broth

Moderate-Carb
- Dandelion greens
- Jicama
- Kale
- Turnip greens

MODERATE ALKALINE

Low Carb
- Arugala
- Asparagus
- Basil
- Broccoli
- Cauliflower
- Celery
- Chives
- Collard greens
- Endive
- Green Cabbage
- Lettuce
- Mustard greens
- Peppers (hot)
- Pumpkin
- Radishes (red, white)
- Cabbage
- Spring greens
- Tomato
- Turnips
- Watercress

Moderate-Carb
- Artichoke
- Garlic
- Green beans
- Okra
- Squash (winter)
- Soybeans

MILDLY ALKALINE

Low Carb
- Bell peppers
- Bok choy
- Brussels sprouts
- Eggplant
- Herbs and spices
- Mushrooms
- Pickles (not sweetened)
- Squash (summer)
- Zucchini

Moderate-Carb
- Beets
- Carrots
- Leeks
- Onions (red, white)
- Peas
- Red cabbage

FRUIT

HIGHLY ALKALINE

Moderate-Carb
- Cantaloupe
- Melons, other
- Watermeleon
- Mango
- Papaya
- Pineapple

Low-Carb
- Berries

MODERATE ALKALINE

Moderate-Carb
- Apriot
- Avocado
- Lemon
- Lime

MILDLY ALKALINE

Low-Carb
- Coconut, fresh
- Olives

Moderate-Carb
- Grapefruit

Secret #10
Digestive Fire

"It's all fun and games until your metabolism slows down."

UNKNOWN

There are Three Treasures in Chinese Medicine: Jing, Qi and Shen. I've mentioned a couple thus far and in this secret, I will share the Cliff Notes version of these concepts. I say Cliff Notes because these are fundamental concepts in Chinese Medicine that are rich and deep.

- Jing is loosely referred to as our "essence". Consider it a genetic inheritance of your DNA that influences how you age and reproduce.

- Qi is loosely translated to 'life force' or 'energy' that is part of everything that is alive. A person's health is influenced by the quality, quantity and balance of Qi.

- Shen is loosely translated as "spirit", which is housed in our Heart and emanates as the light from our eyes.

Ron Teeguarden of Dragon Herbs uses the analogy of a candle, where Jing is the wax, Qi is the flame that flickers from the candle and Shen is the light from the flame. When we live fast and hard by overindulging in harmful substances, not sleeping or eating well, overworking, overextending ourselves sexually, stressing, or experiencing chronic illness, we start to deplete our "genetic bank account" or burn the wax from the candle more than quickly. We show signs of aging more rapidly because we deplete our Jing. We also show signs of aging when our Shen, or light, is dim, dull or disturbed from an unhealthy lifestyle.

The good news is that we can buffer the use of our Jing by cultivating our Qi and we can let our Shen shine through mindfulness and healthy emotional processing. There are many practices that can help preserve our Jing, cultivate our Qi and clear our Shen. In this secret, we will focus on cultivating our Qi. The quality of your Qi relies on the quality of breath and nourishment.

The Chinese character for Qi shows steam rising from a pot of cooking rice. In order to maintain health, we need our metabolism to circulate and activate fuel throughout our bodies. When we digest ice, cold or raw foods, we douse our internal fire. We need to keep our core warm so our digestive fire is strong and our organs receive an abundant supply of oxygen nutrient rich blood. We need to protect our Qi, which will in turn protect our other two treasures, our Jing (essence) and Shen (spirit).

There is a belief in Chinese Medicine that heat is for the living and cold is for dead people. It sounds morbid, I know, but when we keep our core warm, we can experience more endurance, stronger immunity, less back pain, and stronger sexual vitality. Cold saps your Jing and Qi's strength.

Ingesting warming drinks and foods and keeping our core warm with clothing, heat packs or a Harimake are great ways to do so. The Harimake was developed by the Japanese as a wide band of soft wool or flannel cloth worn around the waist, which protects our source of Qi that influences our digestion, energy, sexual vitality and immunity. Wearing a Harimake helps to hold the energy in this area and protects you from stress, exhaustion and illness, especially if you work outside or on your feet all day, or in an over-air conditioned environment, if you have low energy or low back pain or are constantly exposed to cold air.

These methods to preserve heat in our core help alleviate issues with pain, digestion, elimination and fertility.

Action Step: *Choose one way you plan to keep your metabolism high, whether it's reducing cold or raw consumption, increasing spices, dressing warmer, or using heat packs.Get some sun. Allow yourself to bask in its warmth and soak in Vitamin D, the sunshine hormone. Vitamin D is also an amazing serotonin-booster, getting the happy hormones flowing. It also supports your digestive fire. Okinawans spend time outside each day, which allows them to have optimum vitamin D levels all year round*.*

_____

_____

_____

*Okinawa is one of the six designated Blue Zones on the planet where the majority of people live to the age of 100 (centenarians) through lifestyle practices. The Blue Zones is a great resource on healthy aging.

Secret #11
All Roads Lead to the Face

"The face is the soul of the body."

LUDWIG WITTGENSTEIN

Whenever I meet a new patient, I intend to demystify acupuncture by educating them on how this ancient art and science works. I have a chart in my office that artfully depicts where the meridians travel along the body. I explain to my clients when they relax on my table that each meridian connects to an organ system and travels along the body like train tracks, in which Qi and Blood travel and deliver nutrients and oxygen to these organ systems. It takes approximately 20 minutes for Qi to travel along the meridians (I refer to it as the "Qi train") in a circular network.

When we experience imbalance or dis-ease, it is because our Qi becomes stagnant and/or deficient. This happens when external or internal evils block the flow of Qi. You can think of it as a hose with running water that gets kinked. On one end, pressure and stagnation is building and on the other end, little or no energy or flow is happening. Acupuncture and acupressure help to address the blockages in the train tracks or "un-kink" the hose.

The meridians travel all over our bodies and there are some studies that link them to our fascia. The fascia is the tissue that wraps all around our joints, bones, ligaments, tendons and muscles, much like a Saran Wrap encasing. It is the connective tissue that you may see when cutting into a steak (apologies to my vegetarians and vegans reading, it helps to visualize because fascia is not often referenced in Western medicine). Studies have shown that the fascia network is interconnected with blood vessels and nerve endings. This network acts as an electrical highway, conducting signals and messages to our entire body. When someone has a wrinkle in their face, I explain that a wrinkle is a result of a repetitive expression that causes a crinkle in our fascia. Gua Sha, facial rolling and cupping are great modalities for your face and body that help to relieve muscle tension, stimulate lymph and circulation, release lactic acid and smooth out adhesions in our fascia.

The face serves as a microcosm of the body, where every organ is represented. Many meridians start or end on the face. When I talk about secrets to Glow Up, I am referring to the radiant energy that is reflected in your skin, face, body, mind and spirit from the health of your Jing, Qi and Shen. Therefore, just know that when your organs are healthy, your body is healthy, which reflects on your skin, face and spirit as well. In fact, when you activate circulation via acupressure on your face, it promotes total body health as well and vice versa. Here is a picture of the meridians and in the next secret we will go over some acupressure points you can press on to activate total health, beauty and wellness.

Action Step: *at home – continue to practice lymph brushing and facial Gua Sha daily. Book a session with a licensed practitioner in your area to treat your body to acupuncture or cupping.*

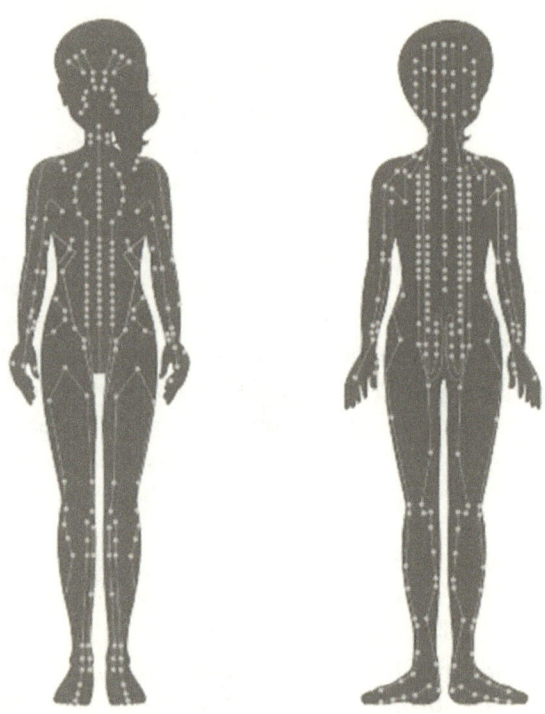

Meridians are located along the body and connect to an organ system. I often describe these pathways as "train tracks". The "Qi train" carries nutrients from food and oxygen (energy) throughout the body. This transport cycle takes approximately 20 minutes to travel through all of the 14 meridians in your body. Acupressure helps to free the Qi train. Where there is more flow, there is more glow!

Secret #12
Magic Buttons

"What you think about activates a vibration within you."

ABRAHAM HICKS

Our bodies are miraculous machines. They can reveal so much about our tendencies and patterns and it takes a considerable amount of time to change our bodies. The one thing that can change in an instant is our face. Our faces are the most dynamic parts of our bodies that reveal so much wisdom.

Acupressure is a modality that can release tension, boost circulation and promote healing in our bodies. We have a minimum of 365 acupressure points on our body. Studies have shown that acupuncture points are frequently described as having distinct electrical properties. These properties include increased conductance, reduced impedance and resistance, increased capacitance, and elevated electrical potential compared to adjacent non acupuncture points.*.

Reduced resistance means there is more flow in these areas.

I love to press on acupressure points on my client's faces over the warmth of a hot towel. I also love to press acupressure points on my own face and state affirmations to solidify a thought and connect it to my body. Emotional Freedom Technique, or EFT, is a process where tapping on acupressure points while vocalizing thoughts can release trapped emotions or blocked Qi. Because I work on faces so much in a quiet dark room, I press on points and silently affirm intentions of healing. When I perform my own skincare routine, I press on these points and say the following:

- **Yintang** I am calm and at peace
- **Gallbladder 14** I am clear on what I desire, what works for me and what does not
- **Taiyang** I am relaxed and willing to be flexible
- **Bitong** I am open to clarity, love and joy
- **Large Intestine 20** I release what does not serve me to make room for what does
- **Small Intestine 18** I am cheerful, healthy, happy and wise
- **Stomach 7** I am confident in my abilities, skills and expertise
- **Stomach 6** I trust that I have all I need to thrive
- **Stomach 5** I love myself unapologetically
- **Stomach 4** I am open to receiving as much as I give
- **DU 24** I am creative, abundant and I invite miracles into my day
- **Ren 24** I am fiercely protective of my energy

You can even create your own affirmations. Abraham Hicks, an inspirational speaker and author, states "hold a thought for just 17 seconds and The Law of Attraction sets in...hold a thought for 68 seconds and things move; manifestation begins. Pressing on acupressure points where flow is in least resistance while stating your desires is a practice that has helped me yield significant results – from healing pain to creating opportunities in my business.

Action Step: *What is something you desire? Hold that thought for just a little over a minute and press on any of these magic buttons below to activate your desire.*

*https://www.ncbi.nlm.nih.gov/pmc/articles/PMC2386953/#idm-139667432084720title

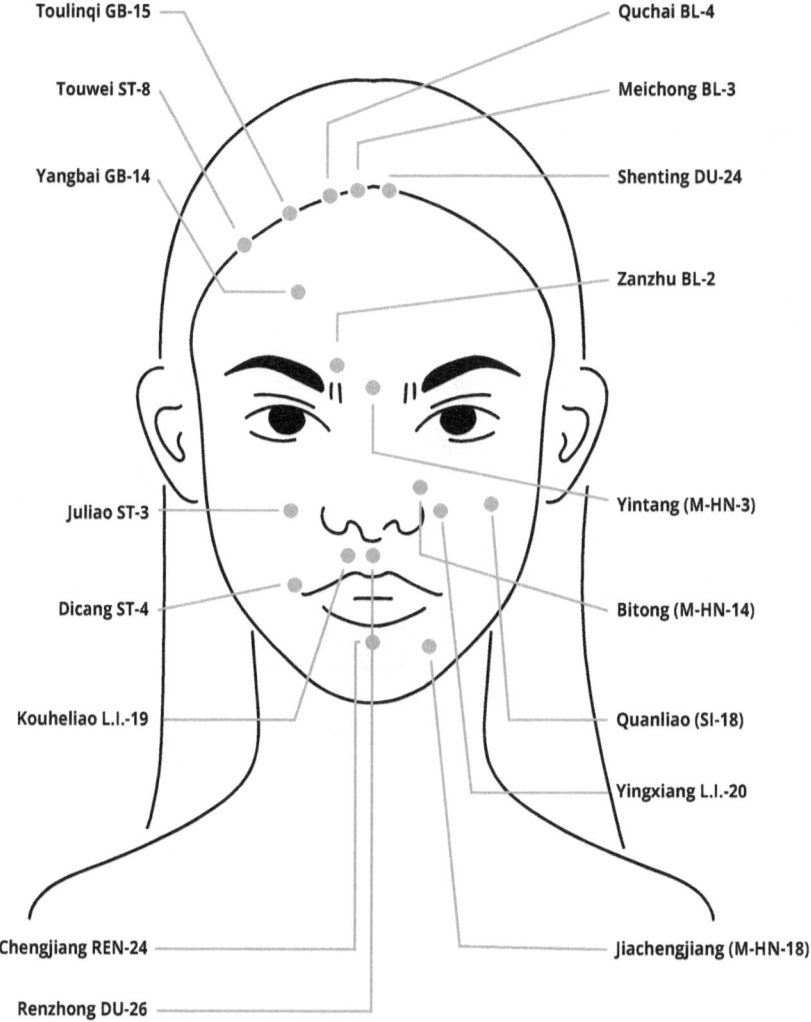

Secret #13
Twerk it

"Nothing happens until something moves."

ALBERT EINSTEIN

I used to despise the word "exercise". I would associate it with high intensity, obsessive tracking of numbers and obligation. Then one day I joined a yoga class where the instructor cued "Move as yourself. Move your body in the way it is designed to express who you are." At first I thought "what is she talking about?". And then, as if my soul was called from its slumber, I started to flow in a rhythm and method that was my own to the music. In the class, each person was given a suggestion to explore a shape and also encouraged to do their own thing, to move in the way their body wanted to move.

Since then, I've reframed the word exercise to mean movement. Everyday, I ask my body what it needs. If I'm tired, I explore gentle movements, like walking or gentle stretching. If I'm looking to build strength,

I lift weights. If I'm looking to burn excessive energy and get my heart pumping, I hop on my Peloton for great music, inspiring guidance and to sweat. If I'm having a slower morning, I practice what I call "lazy yoga" in bed. I do a series of Yin Yoga postures in my bed and hold each posture for 3-5 minutes. I lay in butterfly, twist on each side, ½ saddle on each side, pigeon on each side and forward fold.

My favorite method of movement is dancing. I find that many people either feel they are a great dancer or not so great dancer. It is my belief that everyone can be a great dancer but if you believe that you are not one, you suppress the opportunity to express and move your body as yourself. I invite you to turn on some tunes and just let yourself groove. Let the music you enjoy move you. Dancing is one of the ways you can experience freedom, creativity and power by owning who you are. If you're still feeling apprehensive about it, take a quick tutorial on YouTube. It can be fast, slow, simple or complex and in any style - just get moving! Once you start flowing, your energy will increase and your whole body will glow.

Action Step: *Choose a 5 to 20 minute movement ritual you will practice that is **out of your comfort zone** for the next 7 days.*

Secret #14
Park It

"Flying starts from the ground. The more grounded you are, the higher you fly."

J.R. RIM

When my husband and I first moved to Indiana, we weren't so sure if we planned to stay. We spent many years living "one foot out the door", searching for a new home in a new state. I even hired an astro-cartographer to place our astrology charts over a map and tell us where we should move for optimal happiness and success. In the midst of our search, I moved my practice from location to location, never finding a place to park to allow my practice to truly flourish.

When our daughter was born, we knew we had to set up a solid foundation for her. We decided to give Indy a chance, so I signed a 3 year lease for an office space and six months later, we bought a home. In less than one year, I grossed the highest monthly income practicing acupuncture and skincare since living in Indy for the past 8 years, even in the midst of a pandemic. I hired another team member and expanded my retail and service offerings. I grew my client base and increased my social media following. How did I do this?

I parked.

When you make a decision to plant roots and set your foundation, the next natural progression is growth. It's the same concept when yogis say "root to rise". When you set up solid roots in your postures, you can achieve more lift in your branches.

Action Step: *Ask yourself:*

> *Is there an area in your life that you feel scattered or unsettled?*
> *What would you like to grow that needs a solid foundation?*
> *What decisions do you need to make in order to rise?*

Not sure where to start? Here's a tip: get out in nature. The Japanese have a practice called "shinrin-yoku", known as forest bathing. Spend a day with the trees. Notice how they grow towards the light. Soak up the grounding energy of their roots, the centering energy of their trunks and the lifting energy of their branches.

Secret #15
Presence

"If you are depressed you are living in the past.
If you are anxious you are living in the future.
If you are at peace you are living in the present."

LAO TZU

One of the most powerful resources you own is your presence. To give something your full attention is to cultivate true and deep connection. Connection is the result of being fully present – whether that is being connected to the earth, yourself, someone else or a higher power. I always share with my clients that the past and future are not here and the only moment that is truly guaranteed is now. That means to be fully present is to be fully living in the now.

I invite you to explore what that means to you. One of the tools I use to cultivate presence for myself is sensory awareness. I tune into each of my senses to understand what information my mind, body and spirit are taking in in my current environment. I notice and observe the sounds around me, what my eyes are witnessing, what smells are circulating, what taste lingers on my breath and what my body is feeling – both physical sensations and emotions. I often share with my clients that an emotion is never wrong, it simply is an alert signal that serves as information that something is off and we need to express it (emotion is energy in motion), otherwise we create suppression, which will ultimately lead to over-expression. Remember that kink in a hose? On one side there is not much energy (suppression) and on the other there is pent up energy (over-expression). According to Chinese Medicine, there is a healthy expression and transformation of each emotion:

> From fear to curiosity, courage and wisdom
> From anger to benevolence, compassion, forgiveness and patience
> From anxiety to love and presence
> From worry to trust and faith
> From grief to gratitude

In order to process emotions in a healthy way, we need to really feel them. We need to go through them. We need to be present, attentive and observant to these signals that exist for our survival. Anytime we resist feeling these emotions, we "kink our hoses" and we get stuck in pain. Tune into the wisdom of your body by observing your senses. Allow yourself to get deeply connected to your body's intelligence by noticing what the feeling feels like in your body. Where is it located? What shape is it? What color? Is there a movement or sensation? Be fully present with it and breathe into it. Invite healing and transformation. It may not happen immediately, but the more you practice being fully present, the more your heart's radiance will glow.

Action Step: *Set a time to perform a 5 min body scan from head to toe. Check out the Body Scan visualization on www.mariannetalkovski.com/glowup for a guided experience.*

Take note, what sensations where prevalent?

What emotions came forth?

___

___

___

___

___

___

___

___

___

___

___

Secret #16
Chill Pill

"You cannot always control what goes on outside. But you can always control what goes on inside."

WAYNE DYER

I've talked about emotions serving as alerts to signal us of any threats to our survival. Fear is an emotion that is designed to protect us and keep us safe from danger. The universal function of fear is to reduce or avoid harm. When you perceive a real or imagined physical or psychological threat, your body knows it. Your chin quivers. The hair on the back of your neck stands up or goosebumps appear on your arms. Your heart races. You experience shivers down your spine. You may even pee your pants (no judgment!).

In Chinese Medicine, the Kidneys govern fear. Fear can range on a spectrum between trepidation, nervousness, anxiety, dread, desperation, panic, horror and terror*. In some instances, fear can save our lives. However, living in constant fear can be paralyzing and traumatizing. It can be limiting and depleting. You may be fearful of failure, judgements, bankruptcy, never finding love, abandonment, the public, the government, illness or death, aging, or any other phobias. As mentioned previously, each emotion serves as a signal, alerting us to pay attention, and there is a healthy expression of each emotion. When it comes to fear, the healthy expression is courage and wisdom.

I remember watching Cesar Milan, The Dog Whisperer, coach a family on how to get their chihuahua to behave. He instructed the dog owners to be the alphas of the relationship, which he advised would require them to be in a position of power. What he shared next has stayed with me ever since. He taught these dog owners that the most powerful people in the room are the people who are the most calm and assertive. It is through this state of being that one can lead. Now if you are being attacked by a predator, I am not suggesting that you go into a Zen-like trance. What I am suggesting is that when you are calm, you can make better decisions and take assertive action.

Case and point, in July 2015 I was traveling to visit a client during inclement weather, driving 65 mph, when I hydroplaned. All of a sudden in my peripheral vision, I saw a semi and knew we were going to collide. My first thought was "am I going to die?" I immediately responded "NO!". From there, I surrendered to the moment. Because I was eerily calm, my body did not tense up when the semi hit me, or when I triple turned into a median, or even when I felt the impact of the airbags. My car was totaled, yet luckily, I walked away unscathed. Twenty minutes before my wreck, I had stopped for gas and had applied a calming essential oil blend to my pulse points. I know without a doubt that it was my calm manner plus divine intervention that helped me to maneuver away from the semi, so instead of being T-boned, the driver hit my headlight instead. It was my calm demeanor that saved me from panic and allowed me to act quickly to choose to survive.

There is so much more I can say about fear, but I ultimately want to leave you with this: explore what helps you stay calm and gets your nervous system into a parasympathetic state (rest and digest) and out of the sympathetic state (fight or flight). Take that as your Chill Pill. For me, some of my Chill Pills are listening to relaxing music, not watching the news, wearing essential oils, getting bodywork done, limiting stimulants and getting quality sleep. I protect my peace. Many of my clients rely on acupuncture or facials as their Chill Pill. Commit to discovering what your version is and take it on a consistent basis so you can lean on your courage and wisdom over your fears.

Action Step: *Take a minute to notice what areas in your life you feel tied to obligations and the thoughts associated with them. Write them down. Once you have your list, ask yourself, why do I choose to do this? Is it because I want to or I have to do it? If the answer is "I have to do it" ask yourself "what will happen if I don't do it? What am I afraid of?" Some examples are: "I have to stay connected on Facebook. I have to work this hard. I have to take these phone calls. I have to continue this friendship."*

Action Step: *Make a list of 10 Chill Pills you can take on a regular basis to protect your peace.*

_____

_____

_____

*Source: Atlas of Emotions

Secret #17
Being

"Be the change that you wish to see in the world."

MAHATMA GHANDI

Who you are being is what you are getting.

>Being joyful? You'll get joy.
>Being stressed? You'll get stress.
>Being aware? You'll get awareness.
>Being visible? You'll get seen.
>Being still? You'll get stillness.
>Being generous? You'll get generosity.
>Being closed to receiving? You'll get lack of receptivity.

Another way to look at this is "what are you getting"? Then ask yourself who are you being to get that.

It's a simple secret, yet profound. Being authentic and true to what you feel and who you are is an act of self-love that serves everyone.

Our being-ness is our glow.

Action Step: *Open to your inner wisdom:*

What are you getting or experiencing in your life?

Who are you being to get that?

Currently in my work / relationships / health / finances / self-care I am experiencing....

I am experiencing this because I have been choosing...

I have been choosing this because I feel...

I feel this because I think....

_____

_____

_____

_____

_____

_____

Secret #18
The Bouncer

"No" is a complete sentence."

ANNE LAMOTT

In Chinese Medicine, there is an organ called the Pericardium that serves as the Heart Protector. I like to refer to it as "The Bouncer". It is an organ of discernment and boundary, because it filters what should come in energetically and what should not. I've noticed that many of my clients feel comfortable and safe to express their vulnerabilities in session, and then they return to their fast-paced lives and environments, feeling soft and open. What I've discovered is that they need to be "buttoned or zipped back up" before leaving my office so they are not feeling so blissful that they experience assaults to their heart.

Here's an experiment: Because we are all energetic beings that are divine expressions of love and light, start to notice when you are around someone if you dim or boost your light around them. If you dim your light, why is that? When you boost your light, take note - what is it about this person that inspires you to boost your light?

I encourage you to pay attention to what dims your light or steals your joy. Relationships can give us so much information about where we need to protect our peace and where we feel supported. Imagine you have a bouncer guarding your heart with a velvet rope. Only love is permitted through. Anything else can lovingly stand on the other side.

Action Step: *Scribe from your heart:*

What dims your light or steals your joy? What is no longer permitted to occupy space in your heart?

What boosts your light? What would you like to experience more of in your life?

What can you say no to that would bring you more joy?

_____

_____

_____

_____

_____

_____

Secret #19
2 Way Street

"The key to effective giving is to stay open to receiving."

BOB BURG

One of the benefits of working in my role is that I come across so many generous people in my industry. I meet healers, mothers, fathers, lovers and friends, from all walks of life. I have noticed when givers suffer from being generous with their time, money, energy, and resources, here's why:

- They give with expectation - "if I give this, I will get that"
- They give with conditions - "in order for me to give this, you have to do that"
- They give with obligation - "I have to give my time because she asked me to"
- They give with attachment - "I have to give this to prove I am worthy of love, safety and belonging"

- They give without receiving - "I don't want to owe anyone anything"
- These are just a few examples of how we can block this natural process of love.

Healthy giving starts with an abundant mindset and an authentic, open, receptive heart. Healthy givers / receivers tend to have a glow about themselves that you can't help but notice.

I hear so many stories of how people identify themselves as "the provider, the helper, the caretaker" and they get stuck in expectations, icky sticky conditions, obligations, attachments and lack of receptivity. Their relationships can be co-dependent, or there is an empathic-narcissistic dynamic that is toxic, depleting and muddy. This can show up as resentment on our faces and in our energy.

But guess what? We are all creators of our destiny and we can choose to be healthy in our generosity.

Should you give your time, money, energy, resources or heart, give because you want to, not because you feel you owe someone something or you expect something in return. Be a healthy giver. Give what you can and what you have, nothing more, nothing less. Give and be open to receive the energy you share in return. The two way street is a healthy rhythm and flow of life. Remember, the more there is flow in your life, the more there is glow in your life.

Action Step: *Spend the next week offering and receiving compliments, hugs, and support. When someone offers you something, say thank you before accepting or rejecting the offer. Notice if you feel guilty receiving or* *if you feel the need to over compensate by over giving.*

List 10 ways you offer or will offer contribution in a healthy way:

How will you be a healthy giver? How will you be open to receiving? What support or help will you ask for? How will your life change with this level of help or support?

_____

_____

_____

_____

_____

_____

_____

_____

_____

_____

_____

_____

Secret #20
Let Go, Let Flow

"When you let go, you create space for better things to enter your life."

UNKNOWN.

In 2015 I was on a mission to grow my coaching practice. A couple of years later, upon speaking with a colleague and friend, I was asked, if you really truly want this, how are you going to fit this into your already full life? That question struck me because I discovered that I could not answer her.

I decided if I were to truly be successful, I would need to create the space to make this happen. I had to carefully assess what could stay in my life and what had to go. My mantra was "let go, let flow". I focused on dropping the weight, burdens, grievances, obstacles, busy work and takers that were occupying space in my life, instead of adding value to it. I cannot emphasize enough how letting go feels light. Because I've been aligned with my passion, I feel my energy has increased with every yes and no I've stated with conviction.

Action Step: *You won't grow unless you let go.*

What would you like to invite into your life?

In order to make room for this to come in, who and what can you let go of?

Where can you grow in your life when you stop holding on?

___

___

___

___

___

___

___

___

___

Secret #21
The Golden Nugget

"The mind that opens to a new idea never returns to its original size."

ALBERT EINSTEIN

There is a trick I have adopted that helps me stay present, open and curious in conversations, whenever I get coached, when I'm in a learning environment and even when I'm in a challenging situation. That trick is what I call "The Golden Nugget".

For the majority of my 30s I was not only educating my patients and clients in the treatment room, but I was also educating for a major skincare company where I traveled to many spas and visited with owners, estheticians, front desk staff, massage therapists, etc. During trainings, I would go over product knowledge, retailing and massage techniques with anyone that attended. In my travels, I noticed that the most successful people shared specific common qualities:

They listened with a beginner's mind.
No matter how new or seasoned the professional was, they listened to the material as if hearing it for the first time. They listened with openness and curiosity, inquiring "what can I learn from this information?". They were in full discovery and curiosity instead of approaching each presentation as if they already knew it all.

They were passionate and enthusiastic.
They continued to seek inspiration and show up with infectious joy about their craft. When they discovered something new or of value, they shared it, as if it was treasured gold.

They were open to self-reflecting.
After the trainings I invited them to reflect and share what they would takeaway from the session. That takeaway was The Golden Nugget.

After facilitating this literally over a thousand times, I've adopted the same practice in general, in my life. I can't tell you how many Golden Nuggets I've collected over the years that have helped me heal, grow and transform.

Some big examples of my Golden Nuggets are:

- After two decades of spending thousands of dollars and hours learning from teachers, I learned that I no longer needed to keep investing in "gurus" to teach me what is already inside of me.

- I discovered that I constantly held myself back by thinking I wasn't ready or enough, whether it was my physical appearance, my credentials, my experience or my personality. I realize now that I have everything I need working to connect and serve, that I am ready and the time is now to put myself out there and serve.

- I realized that always looking for validation and recognition outside of myself is disempowering. In order for me to feel fulfilled, whatever I am seeking I need to give to myself.

- I learned that I can only go so far with no support and that in order for me to grow, I need a team behind me that aligns with my values and mission. Those who do not align with me will block my flow and with that discovery, I get to practice the art of letting go of who is not in alignment in order to invite who is in alignment with me, my values and my work. It's not easy, but it's for the greater good of all.

These are profound Golden Nuggets that I've discovered over the years, and I find them in simple moments as well. Ever since I have adopted this practice of inviting the Golden Nugget to appear, my life is filled with curiosity, inquisitiveness and delight. I'm not suggesting to listen with the intent that you have an agenda to get something out of a conversation; I am suggesting to listen with openness, curiosity and wonder versus skepticism, doubt, apathy or ego. Openness, curiosity and wonder contribute to a glowing countenance and people can feel that when you listen with that intention.

Action Step: *Now it's your turn.*

What's one Golden Nugget you are taking away from this book? What's one Golden Nugget you've picked up in conversation or journaling today? Write your discoveries into existence here:

Secret #22
The Bamboo Tree

"Notice that the stiffest tree is most easily cracked, while the bamboo or willow survives by bending with the wind."

BRUCE LEE

Have you ever seen a bamboo tree grow? It's no secret that bamboo is incredibly flexible, sustainable and regenerative. It can grow very quickly during rainy season, with much of the growth occurring underground. It can also withstand a variety of weather conditions. In Chinese Medicine, it is characterized as the energy of Yin Wood. Wood is the element that represents ambition and drive, achieving goals, getting things done, making decisions and leadership. Yang Wood can be thought of as typical Type A personalities, where hustling and climbing the proverbial ladder is the focus and there's no stopping you or getting in your way. Yin Wood is a softer version, where flexibility is just as important as focus. Bamboo is a tree that will continue to grow towards the light, while also pivoting and turning when necessary. Be like bamboo. Stay grounded in your values while also being adaptable to change. Change is the only predictable constant in life and in order to be resilient, we must be flexible and bend. When we are rigid, we become stuck, which blocks our flow and ultimately blocks our glow.

Action Step: *Take a moment here to reflect what is one area of your life that you can be more flexible vs rigid? Career? Relationships? Money? Love? Sex? Family? Purpose?*

_____

_____

_____

_____

_____

_____

_____

_____

_____

_____

Secret #23
The Divine Download

"There is a divine message hidden behind every experience life brings you--both the positive and negative experiences."

AMMA

Have you ever had a night where you woke up at 3 am and couldn't get back to sleep? You toss and turn and try to turn your brain off, but the thoughts keep coming...

When this happens to me, I've discovered that I need to let the thoughts flow. I settle into stillness and listen. Then, all of sudden a thought appears. Loud and clear. Or subtle and clear. But it's there, giving me guidance. I call this the Divine Download.

Now you don't have to wait until you are disturbed out of your sleep to access your Divine Download. It can come to you while you are taking a shower. It can arrive while you are sitting in traffic. It can appear during meditation or practicing Secret #27.

During my Deep Coaching certification*, I learned a technique to drop into deep reflection. It requires conversing with the body's three intelligences: the mind, gut and heart.

- Start with what is at the forefront of your mind. Connect with the pressing thought and the story behind it. Explore the entire story and the thoughts associated with that story. Be the observer of your thoughts and witness what they are creating in your life. Take your time really getting all of your thoughts out.

- Next, connect with your gut. What is your body telling you? What do you feel from these thoughts? What sensations are coming up? How long have these sensations been living in your body? What are you experiencing from them? How have you been transmitting them out into the world through your body?

- Then, access your heart space and listen to what it reveals. Deep down what does it want you to know? What do you know to be true?

- Finally, allow the conversations of these three intelligences to integrate by speaking to one another. Whatever realization that comes from this is your Divine Download.

- Note: this excerpt is an abbreviated version of the process.

Action Step: *listen to the meditation on Divine Download at www.mariannetalkovski.com/glowup for a guided version and record your realization here:*

*Deep Coaching - The Deep Coaching approach is a new paradigm of coaching designed by my coach and mentor Leon VanderPol to meet the needs of all those who are ready to embrace the fullness and magnificence of who they are.

Secret #24
The Garden

"We are all gardeners, planting seeds of intention and watering them with attention in every moment of every day."

CRISTEN RODGERS

I'm not much of a gardener but I happen to love plants. Since opening my wellness spa in Indianapolis, I set an intention that my clients would feel serene in this sanctuary of peace. I wanted to incorporate elements that would boost their Qi. As mentioned previously, the quality of Qi is dependent upon the quality of your food and oxygen intake.

One of the elements I chose in my space was to sprinkle a variety of houseplants that were air purifying in the space. I was not naturally inclined to have a green thumb; however, I took what I learned from Taoist practices and observed nature. I would watch the conditions of the plants that would impact their ability to grow – sun, water, temperature, air and their environment. I observed when the top soil was dry how they were thirsty for water. When their leaves turned brown I knew they were either dehydrated, over-watered or they had specific lighting requirements. When they received optimal care, their stems, leaves and flowers were upright, strong and extra green – as if they had their own glow. When I talked to them while misting them, they responded favorably and produced more leaves or flowers. In this experience, I learned to nurture what I cared about in order for it to grow. I learned to fiercely protect what needed my attention by shielding the plants from insects and adversarial conditions, etc. This is a philosophy that I take with my own self-care practices now as well.

Some of my clients come to me feeling guilty about putting themselves first. They feel undeserving or unworthy, as if everyone else matters more. As a result, they feel depleted, drained, overwhelmed, exhausted and often downright bitter and resentful. I explain that during a plane ride, in the event there is an emergency, we are instructed to put our oxygen masks on first before helping others, otherwise we won't survive and no one else will either. Our survival requires us to fuel ourselves first. A mother cannot breastfeed her child if she has no nourishment. We need to stop this loyalty to martyrdom and tend to our own gardens before we can nurture anyone else.

When my husband tends to our garden, he waters and fertilizes each plant and pulls the weeds. Consider this in all areas of your life. Think about your relationships. What do you want to grow? What needs attentive care? How can you fiercely protect it? What weeds need to be pulled? I've discovered that weeds can manifest in the form of a variety of toxic presentations – the news, social media, people and their beliefs and actions, poor nutrition, polluted environments, etc.

Action Step: *The most important garden you will ever tend to is the garden of your mind. Ask yourself:*

How would you need to take exquisite care of yourself?

In what areas of your life do you need to fuel yourself first?

What would you need to think in order to have what you want?

What thoughts are toxic, destructive or poisonous?

_____

_____

_____

_____

_____

_____

_____

_____

_____

Secret #25
Diamond Glow

"A diamond is a chunk of coal that did well under pressure."

HENRY KISSINGER

It's no secret that stress is inevitable, whether we are living in ancient or modern times. Stress is defined in a medical or biological context as a physical, mental, or emotional factor that causes bodily or mental tension. Stresses can be external (from the environment, psychological, or social situations) or internal (illness, emotional or from a medical procedure). Some signs of stress include: feeling depressed or anxious, making poor decisions, having trouble focusing, experiencing overwhelm, brain fog, or poor memory and feeling unmotivated or hopeless.

Eustress is defined as a positive form of stress having a beneficial effect on health, motivation, performance, and emotional well-being. An example of eustress would be a physical workout or a moderately challenging mental exercise, like putting a puzzle together.

Many of my clients come to me dealing with incredible amounts of stress in their lives. Sometimes there is no end in sight, no light at the end of the tunnel or reprieve. Perhaps they can mitigate their stress levels by delegating workload, enlisting a strong support system, getting creative and resourceful about solutions, taking exquisite care of themselves, drawing clear healthy boundaries on what is acceptable and what is not, or taking a healthy break. I also ask them to evaluate who do they want to be on the other side of their stressful event, when all is said and done. I remind them that pressure creates diamonds* and to focus on your purpose (how you want to serve) to help you through.

Action Step: *There are healthy forms of stress, as mentioned above. Notice if you are resilient or depleted when it comes to stressors. If you feel depleted, what would it take for you to come out on top? What would it take to create a diamond from this situation? What would it take to produce them? (Delegate, enlist support, get creative and resourceful, practice exquisite self-care, draw clear healthy boundaries, take a healthy break)*

What kind of person would you have to be in order to produce them?

Answer these prompts:

I want to look back and say I handled this situation with _____ and experienced this as a result _____.

I relieved my stress because I did the following _____.

I am successful because I became this person: _____

I became this person because I thought this: _____

*Diamonds are formed naturally in the earth's mantle under conditions of extreme temperature and pressure.

Secret #26
An Attitude Of Gratitude

"If the only prayer you say is thank you, that will be enough."

ECKHART TOLLE

One of the most expansive uplifting energies one can experience is the expression of gratitude. Whenever I feel down and my spirits are low, I take a moment to get silent and present, have a meeting with my three centers of intelligence (mind, body and heart) to access my Divine Download and listen for my Golden Nugget. Then I shift into gratitude. I express what I'm grateful for in this moment.

Even if I can't think of anything in the moment, I remind myself that there are people on the other side of the planet that have no access to clean water, live in strenuous circumstances and environments, and don't have access to the many resources that I am blessed to have. I state at minimum 10 things and notice a considerable shift in my mood. In the mornings, before my feet touch the floor I express gratitude for having another day of living on this earth. It's a simple free practice that can transform you from feeling stressed to blessed in seconds.

Action Step: *Write 10 things that you are grateful for in this moment. Practice this every day for 10 days straight and witness the cumulative enhancing effects having an attitude of gratitude has on you and your life over time.*

Bonus step: *Write a thank you note to someone and deliver it to them. Remember that sharing is caring, which will not only elevate your mood, but will lift someone else's spirits as well.*

_____

_____

_____

_____

_____

_____

_____

_____

_____

Secret #27
Silence is Golden

"The quieter you become, the more you are able to hear."

RUMI

There was a time that for every waking moment, I had to fill it with music, phone calls, watching videos of courses online, audiobooks and podcasts, or anything else that could occupy my ears. When I turned forty, I started feeling that I wanted to develop my intuitive abilities. I invested in a countless programs and coaching sessions, took classes, participated in experiential exercises and finally discovered a tool that was pivotal to my intuitive abilities. That tool is silence.

I started sitting in silence. I would take a mini-break here or there. Before I had an appointment scheduled, I would arrive a few minutes early to sit in silence. I would pause in conversation instead of leaping in to say my next thought. It wasn't easy at first to shift from always rushing and being on the go to being still, but over time I started realizing how silence adds ease and grace to my day.

Now I start my mornings with a minimum of ten minutes of silence. Since cultivating this practice, I have noticed my day starts off so much more smoothly and I still get the same amount of things accomplished, if not more. I'm not hustling or jumping out of bed and scrambling. I'm not over-exerting myself, depleting my Jing or shocking my nervous system. I'm much more aware of my surroundings and my senses.

And then there's the juice. The juiciness that surfaces from the depths of quietude. It could be an answer, an idea, an affirmation or a realization. It could be a question, a solution, a reminder or an understanding. It could be anything. When I'm silent, I can hear it. It's in the silence that divine messages can appear. When I can hear them, my heart is open, ready and willing to receive them with a soft place to land. To be silent is to listen. When our hearts are open and soft, and we listen to divine messages, there is a light that emanates from our faces. There is a glow that emanates from our soul.

I invite you to start your day with a minimum of 10 minutes of silence. Drink your lemon water with it. Look out your window towards the sky. Then close your eyes and listen to every sound that comes in and let the silence speak to you. Soon enough, you will discover your own messages from the divine. I invite you to squeeze the juice until the last drop.

Action Step: *Sit in silence for 10 minutes for the next 7 days. Observe how your day flows.*

Secret #28
Kiss Yourself

"Do you want to meet the love of your life? Look in the mirror."

BYRON KATIE

I have a daughter who is full of joy and energy. When she was two and a half, one morning I was getting ready for work, going through the motions of washing my face, brushing my teeth and hair, getting dressed, etc., while she was left to play in the living room with her toys and watch Mickey Mouse Club House on tv. When I didn't hear her shuffling with her legos or jumping up and down on the couch to the mystery Mouseketeers, I peeked in on her to check what she was up to. What I saw caught me by surprise...

She had picked up a mirror I had left on a side table next to our couch. She was looking at herself in the mirror. And then she kissed herself.

I melted. And then I scrambled for my phone to catch it on video. I thought "one day she may not feel so good about herself and when that happens, I want her to witness this moment". I thought how funny is it that she was reminding me how to look at myself, even when I teach this stuff!

Wouldn't it be nice if we all looked at ourselves and felt so much love for who we saw that we kissed our own reflection? I mean, that's what we do with a lover, is it not? We kiss them when we see them because we love them. Some may say that kissing yourself is vain or conceited, but I would argue that to not love who you see in the mirror is the root of all insecurity, shame, rejection, doubt, fear, criticism and pain.

I challenge you to put this book down, walk straight up to the mirror and say "I love you" and then kiss yourself. When you love yourself when you see yourself, you elevate humanity because you elevate yourself. Go do it. Do it for yourself. And do it for humanity. Do it every morning and every night. Blow yourself a kiss every time you see your reflection. Even if you don't fall in love with yourself right away, you may find yourself laughing. And laughing, my friend, is the best tip for radiant energy. Laughing is the best way to show your glow, even when no one is watching. Or you never know, a child, friend or friend you haven't met yet may be watching you. What do you want to teach him or her?

Action Step: *Put this book down, walk straight up to the mirror and say "I love you" and then kiss yourself. Vow to blow yourself a kiss every time you see your reflection for the next 30 days. Finally, answer these prompts:*

What are 10 things I love about myself?

What are 10 ways I will show myself I love myself?

A Self-Care Manifesto

When I love myself unapologetically and take care of
myself exquisitely, I don't rely on validation, approval or acceptance
outside of myself.

I drown out the noise, including the voice of my own inner critic.

I recognize my worth and the value I contribute to the world.

When I express myself boldly and freely from my real and raw heart
and speak what's true for me now, I heal and shine and empower
others to do the same.

~Marianne Talkovski

Resources

Visit www.mariannetalkovski.com/glowup for resources on skincare, nutrition, meditation and more!

Acknowledgements

My husband Nate for your unconditional love, support and laughs.

My daughter Jasmine, for teaching me to slow down and smell the flowers.

Daryl Thuroff, my suga D, for always being there with me through thick and thin.

Cathy Riccio, my little Stink, for being brave enough to grow and for sharing your loyal heart of gold.

Amanda Reagan, for your sisterhood and supportive ear. You've always had my back, since we were 12, even through the storms.

Ambre Crockett, my spiritual running buddy, for always keeping it real and showing me love.

Erin Halloran, my soul sister, for being such a positive reflection in my life and reminding me that anything is possible & magical every time we speak.

Samantha Zillig, my Scorpio sis, for giving me endless boosts & pep talks – glad for Marco Polo!

Ivana Siska, for reflecting beauty, power & wisdom back to me & cheering me on.

Lillian Bridges, for teaching me Chinese Face Reading, and loving me like family.

Leon VanderPol, for reminding me that I am a sanctuary of peace.

Susan Hyatt, for teaching me I have a voice, I am a force to smash diet and hustle culture and that self-care is a business strategy. Thank you for believing in me to raise the bar in diversity, equity, inclusion, female empowerment, body positivity and ALL THE THINGS.

Mom, for giving me life and purpose.

Rick, for reminding me where we come from and how much we've grown.

Next Steps

Visit **www.mariannetalkovski.com**

Join the Rebel Beauties community at **www.facebook.com/groups/rebelbeautiesrule**

Post your favorite tip on Instagram and tag @mariannetalkovski with hashtag #RadiantEnergySecrets

Subscribe to the Humanity Speaks: The Human In The Mirror podcast featured on iTunes & Spotify to hear stories mixed with Chinese Face Reading and messages on what each guest believes humanity needs most.

About Marianne

Marianne is a licensed acupuncturist, esthetician, Transformational Coaching MASTER CERTIFIED Coach, Certified Deep Transformational Coach and Bare Coach in Training. She guides her clients to find their most authentic expression of beauty in radical self-acceptance, regardless of the messages our culture has inundated us with to consume, perfect, compare, critique and feel less than enough.

Her foundational teaching is that by investing in your self-care and owning who you are, the ultimate act of healing, love, connection and beauty is activated not only in one's soul, but for all humanity. She stands for all humans to raise their voices against forces of oppression, especially diet culture.

Since becoming a mother, Marianne is determined to create a world where her daughter knows what self-acceptance, self-care, self-healing and self-love looks like. She guides all walks of life through these tenets in her signature programs Picture Ready Skin, New You By Design and Get Radiant Energy. Since committing to this message, she has never felt more radiant, happy, healthy and powerful.

Thank you!

Thank you so much for taking the time to read this book. It is my intention that you take what resonates with you and put it into practice so you can glow as the radiant human being that you are.

With love,

Marianne

www.ingramcontent.com/pod-product-compliance
Lightning Source LLC
Chambersburg PA
CBHW021954290426
44108CB00012B/1070